CREATE A SAFE SPACE

*An Inspirational Guidebook for Yoga Teachers
Who want to Further Serve their Students*

Gudjon Bergmann

Create a Safe Space

Copyright © 2010 by Gudjon Bergmann

ISBN 978-1453890790

Table of Contents

INTRODUCTION: CREATE A SAFE SPACE

"Put your heart, mind, intellect and soul even to your smallest acts. This is the secret of success."
- Swami Sivananda

Dear yoga teacher,

This guidebook is written for you. It doesn't matter whether you have just completed a yoga teacher training, are still in training, or have taught yoga successfully for years, you should be able to benefit from reading the following pages.

For the novice, this book should provide friendly advice, based on my years of experience, advice that can save both time and effort; and for the experienced yogi, the book can serve as a sounding board for comparing ideas and teaching approaches.

The book is not written for any specific style, branch or brand of yoga, but for all yoga teachers, regardless of their background.

The idea of creating a safe space, for both the student and teacher, and for both to prosper and grow, was first voiced in the primary stages of my training as a yoga teacher. It has been my guiding light while teaching thousands of hours of yoga, running a successful yoga studio, training dozens of yoga teachers, raising a family and following my own spiritual path. The advice in this book is based on (1) my *experience*, (2) the *guidance* I have received from my teachers, and (3) my *interaction* with the yoga teachers I have trained. I hope it will be of use to you.

When I ran my yoga studio from 2001-2006, the first sound uttered from most of my students when they entered the studio was a soft sigh, sort of an *"aaahhh…"*, a sound of relief. They had found a safe refuge, a haven, a place where they didn't need to think; they were free from distractions and could leave their worries behind, if even for a moment. This reaction was one of the signs that I had *created a safe space*. I had succeeded.

The great thing about having trained dozens of yoga teachers is that once the training starts, the students begin to ask questions about how to create this safe space, this haven. Their questions are in part what has made this book possible, because I had to explain what I did right and what went wrong along the way.

I have always been humble to the fact that there *isn't one right way to do things*, it isn't *my way or the highway*, but success leaves clues, and I must have done something right because the attendance was rather high, 300-500 visits a week, in a studio that only took a maximum of 20-25 people per class.

The following is a list of what I did to create a safe space. Each item will be explained in a later chapter. The chapters are not prioritized in any particular order, they are brief and to the point, and so is the book, but if used properly it can become a source of inspiration and can be read and re-read as needed.

- Keep your studio clean
- Be punctual and start your classes on time
- Give clear and loud instructions
- Be self-confident and well prepared
- Know anatomy in relation to yoga
- Know the Purpose of a Pose

- Learn to say: "I don't know"
- Relaxation and visualization
- Construct clear boundaries
- Infuse your teachings with your own experience
- Don't give into boredom
- Learn to interpret and teach the philosophical and spiritual aspects of yoga
- Don't use your classes for personal practice
- Deepen your personal practice
- Encourage growth and questioning
- Use marketing with a service orientation
- Practice the ethical guidelines of yoga
- Infuse yoga with modern approaches to create the yoga of the future

Of course more can be done to create a safe space, but these are the ideas and practices I would like to emphasize in a friendly atmosphere. I hope you take some of them to heart, even if you decide not to use all of them.

Gudjon Bergmann
www.gudjonbergmann.com

KEEP YOUR
STUDIO CLEAN

"Opportunity is missed by most people because it is dressed in overalls, and looks like work."
- Thomas A. Edison

Imagine lying on your mat, breathing intensely, feeling good … and then creating a cloud of dust with your exhalation, or, almost fainting at the smell of perspiration, or, seeing grime in every corner of the dressing room, or… you get the picture.

Nobody wants to do yoga poses or meditate in dirty surroundings. The first step to creating a safe space for your students is the appearance of your studio, and I advise you to keep it clean by any means necessary. Before I owned my own studio, I taught in various places such as gyms, workplaces, and other yoga studios, and I remember that I always *made myself responsible* for keeping the rooms I taught in as clean as possible. That often meant I had to go out of my way and do something that I was not being paid to do, such as mop or sweep the floors, but I still made it my responsibility. My primary duty has always been to create a safe, and clean, space for my students, and that has meant cleaning up more than my share of rooms through the years, with joy I must add.

If you run your own yoga studio, you will without a doubt want to create an atmosphere of ease and comfort. Cleanliness is an integral part of that process. My studio was a low budget enterprise and for three years out of the five that I ran it, I cleaned it myself. That meant mopping the floors at least once or twice daily, cleaning the mats two or three times a week depending on traffic, maintaining good air conditioning, cleaning the dressing rooms and restrooms every day, and more. This was hard work, but well worth it. Almost every one of my regulars commented at one time or another on how clean the place was.

Finding joy in cleaning wasn't very hard. While cleaning, I chanted mantras, thought about how my manual labor would benefit my customers, listened to audio programs, listened to music, or transformed the act of cleaning into a moving meditation. With the right attitude the work was a joy, a valuable service, and everyone benefitted from it.

With increased workload and attendance I could no longer clean the way I used to, so I got assistance. It took time to train the people who took over the job and to help them understand the *importance* of keeping the studio clean. I also enlisted the help of other yoga teachers who taught in my studio, and when they understood the importance, they took part in the cleaning if needed, without hesitation, and in the spirit of joyful service.

The job of cleaning is in most societies looked at as a job of low importance, is usually a low paying job, and probably won't rise to any great heights soon. But given how important cleanliness is in our surroundings, we yoga teachers should re-think how we treat those who have the important job of cleaning, and partake in the process if the need arises.

Many people would think of this advice as a no-brainer, thinking that it shouldn't even be in this book, but given some of the yoga places I have visited, both in the USA and Europe, where there has been a distinct lack in cleanliness, the advice is both valid and important.

BE PUNCTUAL AND START YOUR CLASSES ON TIME

"Eighty percent of success is showing up."
- Woody Allen

My rule in relation to time management and teaching is simple: *"If you're on time, you're late!"* That means that if you arrive *just on time* to teach, you have no flexibility. In essence nothing can go wrong, and in addition to that, your mind probably won't settle until halfway through the class.

I have been teaching since 1998 and taught well over six thousand yoga classes, in addition to hundreds of lectures and seminars, and I have *never been late*. That doesn't mean I am better or special. It just means that I have adopted a simple rule of *always being early*.

I have encountered traffic jams, my tire has blown out a few times, I have forgotten all my gear at home and encountered numerous other unforeseen instances, but that hasn't changed the fact that I haven't been late yet. There is a minor downside to this rule. Factoring in these unforeseen circumstances has translated into a lot of waiting time, which most time management experts probably wouldn't find very effective or productive. But, I have used that *downtime* for meditation, contemplation, reading, listening to seminars and preparing for my classes.

You can't buy a reputation, and your behavior precedes you. If you are continually late, it will have an ill effect on your income, your students, and your reputation.

Through my years of practice and teaching I had noticed that *only a few people*, and usually *the same people*, came late to class, and caused unwanted disturbance. I thought to myself that these people were being given unwarranted advantage and decided to set the following rule at my studio:

"Out of respect to the people who arrive on time, the studio doors will be closed and locked when classes start."

Create a Safe Space

I locked the doors and started each class punctually. The result was tremendously positive. The punctual people, *the majority*, were pleased, and if people came late, they either didn't arrive late again or didn't come again at all (very few people quit the studio because of this rule, but some did, and I decided it was worth it). Either way, I thought it was a positive rule, and so did most of my patrons.

The same went for finishing classes on time. I realized that in today's atmosphere you can't *give* people time. Most people are booked solid and complain about lack of time. If you prolong the relaxation or meditation, or continually break the advertised time frame, you aren't benefitting anyone in the long run. If you want to prolong the meditation or relaxation at the end of your class, ask for permission and be sure that no one has to be done on time before you try to *give* your students extra time. In essence I advise you to start and stop on time, and arrive on the premises with time to spare.

GIVE CLEAR AND LOUD INSTRUCTIONS

"Everything becomes a little different as soon as it is spoken out loud."
- Hermann Hesse

Have you ever been in a yoga class where the teacher spoke in such a low voice that the people in the back of the room were continually breaking their concentration and looking towards the front of the room? Did you sense how uncomfortable that can be for everyone? I have attended way too many yoga classes where the teacher was quite good, but the quality of teaching was overshadowed by the fact that he spoke in a low or soft voice, which in turn created an uncomfortable and unsafe space.

The myth of the *yoga voice* is widespread. Speaking softly and slowly, and breathing through the vocal chords in a low voice, has become the *mythical ideal voice* for a yoga teacher. But unless there has been installed a state of the art sound system in the studio, a yoga teacher should speak in a *clear and loud voice*. Clear, direct and vibrant instructions will inject energy into the class, and create a feeling of safety for the students. Speaking loudly works, even if one is trying to create a soothing and stress free atmosphere. I have tried this and tested with dozens of my teacher trainees and hundreds of my students. Trying to create a *yoga voice* sometimes has the opposite effect, creating stress for the students, because they simply *can't hear* what is being said.

All my yoga teacher trainees have been trained to speak *uncomfortably loud*, which simply means that *they* feel uncomfortable about how loud their voice is; their students don't. During training I have also emphasized that everyone should use their own natural voice.

The feedback that each and every one of my teacher trainees has gotten about their initial teaching from their fellow classmates is almost always about the quality of their voice. Their classmates say something like:

"You have a very good voice for teaching yoga"

"I like your voice"

or ...

"I couldn't hear you all of the time"
"Could you speak up next time?"

and so on ...

The voice is the yoga teacher's most important instrument, whether during a physical yoga class, a guided meditation, or in a lecture. I personally recommend that you find a book, an e-class, a personal voice trainer, or all of the above. I have trained my voice with actors and singers and do voice exercises on a regular basis.

Any voice can be trained to some degree and with that in mind I must relate a story. When I was eighteen I recorded a guided relaxation. It had been something that my mom had done and I wanted to give it a try. When I was done recording I played it back to my half-brother who simply responded: "You don't have a good voice for guiding relaxation. If I were you I wouldn't do it again." And I took his advice at first and just stopped recording, but when I became a yoga teacher I simply *had to* do it, I *had to* guide relaxations. Since then I have taught thousands of hours of yoga and recorded dozens of guided relaxation tapes and CD's. I don't have the best voice in the business, but I very often get praise for having a good voice – and that's all training.

Your voice is your primary tool for teaching. Speak up and be sure to train your vocals on a regular basis.

BE SELF-CONFIDENT
AND WELL PREPARED

"As soon as you trust yourself,
you will know how to live."
- Johann von Goethe

Self-confidence is an essential tool for the yoga teacher who wants to create a safe space. It's easy for a student to feel insecure and unsure if the teacher is ill prepared, doesn't seem to know what he is doing, and shows a distinct lack in self-confidence.

Much has been written and said about self-confidence and not all of it good. From the outset I want to make it clear that self-confidence is not arrogance. If you have self-confidence you will trust yourself to take on any task that life hands you, and, to follow your personal *dharma* or path in life. Self-confidence is built from the *inside out* and has little or nothing to do with outside circumstances.

A person lacking self-confidence will recoil from new challenges and eventually get stuck in a rut or back herself into a corner. She will fall prey to negative self-chatter and continuously shy away from her own gifts and talents.

Conversely a person with self-confidence will follow her personal *dharma*, her path in life, choosing to fully develop and enhance her gifts and talents.

Having self-confidence is not about being better than anyone else, it's about becoming the best version of you, and the yogic approach is to serve others with the talents and abilities you are born with and the ones you have become qualified at performing through training.

You must remember that self-confidence is not a fixed way of thinking or acting. It changes all through your life, increases or decreases, depending on circumstances and internal dialogue. You can have a swelling of self-confidence in one area of life, and at the same time, be completely lacking in another area.

For self-confidence to increase you must learn to control your internal dialogue, make plans to further train in your areas of strength, and learn not to be overly sensitive about your weaknesses. Watch out for the words you use when you talk about yourself. You can for example use strengthening words instead of weak ones (for example *do* instead of *try*, *choose* instead of *have to*, *invest* instead of *spend*, *challenge* instead of *obstacle*, *interesting* instead of *irritating* and so on). Posture is also important. Carry yourself with dignity and self-respect.

Being well prepared wins half the battle. If you are knowledgeable about your area of expertise, i.e. you know your yoga poses, are well spoken, and have a good background in the area of yoga philosophy; your preparedness will serve you well.

Having said that, I must add that a person with less knowledge and more self-confidence (which is primarily a way of thinking and acting) will often run circles around a person with more knowledge and less self-confidence; which means that self-confidence has the upper hand to knowledge when it comes to acting in the world. It has been interesting to see many of my star *academic* students struggle with teaching in the real world, while others who are less qualified in the academic field but have more self-confidence, have gone out and positively affected many more people through their teaching.

The key to success in teaching is to have both, that is, be prepared *and* work on increasing your self-confidence. But, despite all the mental preparation, there is no substitute for *facing fears* and *overcoming challenges* in the real world. Experience trumps both knowledge and ways of thinking every time. So if you want to increase your self-confidence as a yoga teacher very fast – go out there, face your fears, and teach as much as you possibly can!

KNOW ANATOMY IN RELATION TO YOGA

"Good for the body is the work of the body, good for the soul the work of the soul, and good for either the work of the other."

- Henry David Thoreau

When I went through my first yoga teacher training in 1998 there was little or no emphasis on anatomy in relation to yoga. The Indian way of slightly exaggerating the benefits of every pose was the primary mode of teaching and the anatomy teacher had no scientific background. This has changed very much in the years since and for the better. Knowing human anatomy in relation to yoga will make any space where yoga postures are taught much safer.

There are quite a few books out now that focus on anatomy in relation to yoga, but the very best material that I have come across is Paul Grilley's DVD *Anatomy for Yoga*. Increased knowledge about bone structure, range of movement, tension and compression, and proportions between body parts, has created understanding and safety in my classrooms and those of my trainees.

Knowing human anatomy is important when interacting with students, because not every*body* is the same. That knowledge changes the approach of the yoga teacher significantly. Teachers who think that *any range of motion* can be attained by *anyone* through practice, and don't take skeletal differences into account, will be more demanding of their students and even judgmental without realizing it (by telling people that they can achieve something that is physically improbable). Being knowledgeable, doing tests on the students and encouraging them to listen to their bodies and never push too far into painful postures – are just some of the things a yoga teacher who wants to create a safe space should do.

This becomes doubly important in relation to injuries. A friend of mine attended a yoga class in the U.K. many years ago. When performing the triangle pose the yoga teacher in the room stepped on his ankle to push his heel down and tore a few tendons and muscles in the process. Thinking that everyone should look the same once a posture is completed was what led to my friend's painful and unnecessary injury.

In relation to the benefits of yoga postures, there is little need to exaggerate. Instead I recommend that you downplay the benefits and use wording like "can help with", "should lead to", "has proven to be beneficial in many cases" and so on, instead of filling people's heads with promises that neither you nor the yoga postures can deliver.

Knowing anatomical basics and postural differences is a key element in creating a safe space for both teacher and student.

KNOW THE PURPOSE OF A POSE

"Our prime purpose in this life is to help others. And if you can't help them, at least don't hurt them."
- Dalai Lama

At the outset of a yoga teacher's career, once he has finished his training and has just begun teaching, he becomes very aware of how *many postures* there are and how *many variations* other teachers are teaching. This can become very confusing and many of my trainees have questioned me time and time again about the difference between this triangle and the other, one variation of this posture versus another, and so on.

My answer is always in the form of a question. I ask my trainees: "What is the primary purpose of this pose?" If the purpose is a spinal twist, how important is the placement of the palm or fingers? If the purpose is a forward bend, how important is the gaze of the eyes? Surely these little improvements can be important at some point in the practice, but one should focus on the *primary purpose of the pose* first, and then add features or teach variations.

When in doubt, ask yourself about the primary purpose of the posture. If you realize that the posture falls into the category of a backbend, forward bend, inverted pose, spinal twist or hip opener, then you can approach the pose with the same attention you would approach other postures within that group.

The real advice here is not to get caught up in the details and all the different approaches and variations. Yes, they can be nice to add once you have mastered the basics, but like an artist you should really *master the basics* before you try to break or bend the rules.

This will create a safe space for you and your students because you will not be too preoccupied with guiding them through every little nuance of a pose, instead focus on the primary purpose and make sure that nobody is injuring themselves in your class. Stick to purpose!

LEARN TO SAY: "I DON'T KNOW"

"If you know that you don't know, that is a great beginning. Then it is possible for you to know."
- Socrates

For some reason, likely because of the spiritual dimension of yoga (which some people misinterpret as priestly or fatherly), quite a few students are prone to put yoga teachers on pedestals, almost worshipping them and gobbling up their every word. This puts unfair pressure on yoga teachers, because students sometimes ask questions about things that there is no way for the yoga teacher to know or answer. I have had people ask me about personal injuries, finances, their love life and even what to think about important issues in their own life. To take the pressure off, yoga teachers must be willing to step down from this imagined pedestal and utter the words *"I don't know"* on a regular basis.

One rule I have followed from the beginning of my teaching career is that if a person comes to me before or after class and asks about a personal injury and doing yoga, I always start with saying "I don't know about you *personally* or your medical history", and then sometimes add that "it depends on this or that". If applicable I talk about general things a person should keep in mind while doing the postures and general rules about certain postures. To further emphasize that I don't know enough about his or her personal condition, I always refer the student to his or her *doctor* or *physical therapist*. I can never know enough about any one particular case or individual to properly advise about yoga postures and personal injuries.

This has been my rule from the beginning and it has served me well. It's not that I don't advise people according to the best of my knowledge at each time; it's just that I don't take on any responsibility that is beyond my capacity or desired role.

Being able to utter the words "I don't know" demands more self-confidence than pretending to know, quoting hearsay, or repeating unsubstantiated claims, because you have to be willing to face the fear of not knowing how people will react when you confess that you don't know. Fortunately I have never had anyone react in a negative way when I have said "I don't know". The opposite is rather the case, i.e. that people respect me for it.

When I started offering yoga teacher training in 2002 I was not very experienced, or not experienced enough many people thought (including myself), but my teacher Yogi Shanti Desai offered to be my backup and my mentor. He said that whenever I couldn't answer something, I should contact him. That gave me the confidence to offer the first teacher training the year after I opened my yoga studio. Yogi Shanti Desai has been my mentor ever since, and when I tell my students that I don't know, I also add "but Shanti might know, let me ask him", and to tell you the truth, sometimes even he doesn't know …

There is also a big difference between opinion and truth. Once something has been established to be true, you can quote it, but when you give your opinion you should always tell people that it's just that, your opinion.

When you learn to say "I don't know" freely and openly, you will also be open to learn from others, even your students. I have often left center stage in my teacher training programs when I have felt that my students knew more than me, and as a result I have always gained knowledge, without losing face.

RELAXATION AND VISUALIZATION

"Lying flat on the ground with the face upwards, in the manner of a dead body, is shavasana. It removes tiredness and enables the mind (and whole body) to relax."
- Yogi Swatmarama

One of the most sacred times in a yoga class is the relaxation period at the end. People who feel safe will surrender completely and feel refreshed and energized after the class. People, who feel unsafe for any reason, will not be able to relax. Sometimes their uneasy feeling will originate on the inside, so you, the yoga teacher, can't do much about it. What you can do, is create the safest space possible and use the methods that are most likely to lead people into a state of relaxation.

In my experience there are infinitely many ways to help people relax; muscle flexing and relaxing, breathing, music, visualization, sound vibrations and more. I don't want to emphasize one method at the cost of another, but I do want to bring my experiences to your attention, both as a student and teacher in this area.

When teaching relaxation you have choices. You can stick with your own way of teaching, your own preferences, or you can try to find a middle ground, a way of teaching that is likely to reach the largest number of people.

Music is one tool that can either facilitate the relaxation or really irritate people. I have found it best to stick to *neutral music*, nothing overly melodic or emotional. I even use the same music most of the time to reinforce the neural pathways. It works beautifully.

To give you an idea of why this can be important, let me relate a story. While I was directing the teacher training in early 2010, I once swayed from this rule of mine and played a piece of flute music that is both melancholy and melodic, and that I personally love relaxing to. Afterwards I asked the class how it made them feel and they were equally divided. Half the class liked the music while the other half didn't like it at all. What surprised me was the level of *enthusiasm* I encountered. The half that liked the music *really loved it* and asked where they could buy the CD, while the other half was *very irritated*, almost downright mad at me for playing it and ruining their relaxation. *That's why* I stick to neutral or low key music. It creates a safer space for everyone involved.

Visualization can have the same effect. Some people love it, others are bothered by it. Let me take two examples.

The first example is about the content of visualizations. Some teachers use the visual image of a beach when trying to induce relaxation. When I visualize a beach, I don't relax, because I don't like lying on the beach. It just reminds me of getting sand in unwanted places. I would much rather get neutral guidance, guiding me towards a warm and safe place, and let my imagination fill in the blanks.

The other example is about emotional work during relaxation. We all know that emotional catharsis can happen spontaneously or facilitated on purpose during the state of relaxation. I always tell my students that emotional blockages can, for no apparent reason, be removed during relaxation, and that this may leave people feeling strange, sometimes sad, sometimes glad. I tell them not to think about it too much, let it go and don't try to find a cause. I have had people start sobbing uncontrollably and even had two women start laughing hysterically after my classes. My reaction is always the same; let them work it out and give general guidance about dealing with emotional catharsis.

Working with emotional issues on purpose can backfire and should always be done with the prior *approval* and *knowledge* of attendees. One guy told me the story of how he was attending a yoga class and the teacher started telling the students to gather their anger, resentment and other bad feelings into balloons during the relaxation. When he told them to let them go, one man in the room sat up and yelled *"NO"*. He simply wasn't ready to let go. This story reminds us that letting go is a *choice* that cannot be forced upon another human being.

One of the most important things a teacher can do during relaxation is to stay still and give people a safe, non-disturbed space. I know too many stories about teachers who become bored during relaxation and either leave the room (which tends to create an unsafe atmosphere) or start gathering their things and tidying up before bringing the group out of relaxation. Don't do that. Just sit still. I always use the relaxation for contemplation or meditation, and send loving, compassionate thoughts to my students. I advise against lying down with the students and relaxing at the same time, you're bound to stay under too long at some point. I remember teaching the day after my son was born. I hadn't slept much and fell asleep during relaxation. That's when I decided that it might not be such a good idea.

My guidance about relaxation is in line with my attitude towards it. Give general guidelines, offer a safe environment, don't talk too much, let the people enjoy the relaxed state once they have entered it, sit still and rejoice when you see your students awaken and enjoy all the benefits that a deep state of relaxation can offer them.

CONSTRUCT CLEAR BOUNDARIES

"Never grow a wishbone, daughter, where your backbone ought to be."
- Clementine Paddleford

Every yoga teacher training I have directed has started with a one or two hour lecture and discussion about *co-dependency* in relation to teaching yoga. Even though co-dependency is a term closely associated with alcoholism, it has been known to permeate a yoga class or two, especially where the teachers have low self-esteem and lack self-confidence.

Co-dependency essentially revolves around the sentence: *"I am not enough."* A co-dependent person will always need another person to validate their worth, their feelings, their ideas and even their existence. This either expresses itself as a need to manipulate and control surroundings; or as a need to bend over backwards to make other people feel good, the reason being that "*I* can't feel good if *you* don't feel good."

How does this affect the yoga class you might ask? Well, I know a yoga teacher who asks for validation after each and every class. He does it with questions like: "Was the class OK? Was I OK? Is there anything I should do differently next time?" Even though it's good to get feedback every now and then, an incessant need for validation shows lack of self-worth. Receive praise graciously, if it is given freely, but don't go looking for it.

Other examples of co-dependency can appear when a person is always running to meet their students every whim: "Could you turn up the heat? Turn down the heat? Not do this or that?" Again, it's alright to attend to the student's needs and wishes *within reason*, but the teacher's job is to create a safe space for *everyone*, and how can he do that if someone else is really running the class and everyone else can see and feel it? Ask yourself this:

"Would I rather be a peach or a coconut?"

Yogi Shanti Desai asked me this question many years ago and I have used it in many of my seminars and all my teacher trainings. Let me explain.

A *peach* is beautiful on the outside, luscious and attractive, but bruises easily and is extremely hard on the inside. A person who is like a peach is always trying to look good and be good to everyone, but is at the same time getting harder on the inside, constantly feeling more bitter and guilty. Telltale sentences would include the classic: "I do everything for everyone else, why doesn't anyone do anything for me?" It's easy to become hard on the inside if you're waiting for the world to repay your kindness quid pro quo. I have met many peaches in the yoga teaching industry, hell I was one; and there are also many peaches in conventional caretaker industries, such as nurses, teachers, kindergarten teachers, and social workers. These are all *good people* trying to make a difference, but unfortunately many of them have put on a mask of gentleness and try to please everyone they meet (which is simply impossible), instead of focusing on the inside first and letting the internal feelings of self-worth and service orientation expand to the outside.

That's where the *coconut* comes in. Hard and un-inviting on the outside, but once you get past that hard shell, you find yourself in a haven of *superb nourishment*. A person that is more like a coconut may not bend over backwards to make sure everyone she meets likes her, but the people she lets through her shell are bathed with the same love and attention that she nourishes herself with on the inside. The coconut is a reservoir. Now ask yourself again:

"Would I rather be a peach or a coconut?"

Personally, I have chosen to be more like a coconut. To lessen the "peachy" effect on my life I have repeated a sentence that my first yoga teacher, Ásmundur Gunnlaugsson, taught me almost ten years ago, and I have taught it in all my seminars and teacher trainings. The sentence goes like this:

"I am not going to like everyone,
not everyone is going to like me,
and that is perfectly OK."

Most people are quick to agree that they are not going to like everyone they meet. It doesn't mean they should be rude; they're just not going to hit it off with every person they meet, that includes their students. What naturally follows is that not everyone is going to like them. That's harder to swallow, but when accepted it makes life so much easier. Then it's just a matter of reminding oneself repeatedly that it's perfectly OK, it's normal and natural.

Once you have completed this self-examination by asking yourself if you are more like a peach or a coconut, you can either fortify your boundaries or build acceptable ones. A student of mine asked if we can't be a blend of the peach and the coconut. Of course we can, we all are. It's not a black and white picture; it's a metaphor that can be used where and if applicable.

This correlates with the learning to say "I don't know" and increasing your self-confidence. Just remember not to get too involved with your students, construct clear boundaries and keep a professional distance.

I remember this one teacher who came to my training, a woman in her fifties, extremely nice and wanting to be that way to everyone. One year after her training finished she called me on the phone with a problem. Evidently one of her male students had fallen in "love" with her and kept bothering her before and after classes, even calling her on her cell phone. I immediately asked her what *she had done* to allow him that kind of access. At first she said nothing, but through introspection she realized that she *hadn't created a professional barrier*, she had continued to be nice to the guy long after he had overstepped his boundaries.

You don't suddenly *find* yourself in a compromising position like that. You give out a *feel*, a *vibe* of sorts, and people can sense how far they can cross into your space. If you appear *too soft*, someone will try to take over your class and boss you around. If you appear *too nice*, someone will try to misuse that in some way.

Do you remember that teacher from high-school who showed weakness and got hammered by the bullies in class? Well, there are bullies in real life too, and they sometimes attend yoga classes. You don't have to stop being nice, just don't show it to everyone and learn to be tough every now and then, add some *yang* to your *yin*.

INFUSE YOUR TEACHINGS WITH YOUR OWN EXPERIENCE

"A man who carries a cat by the tail learns something he can learn in no other way."
- Mark Twain

When you entered your yoga teacher training you had already amassed experience that can be useful to others, and that experience can become doubly beneficial if you combine it with your knowledge of yoga. Instead of trying to imitate others, think about your experience, and find out *which group of people* you are *uniquely qualified* to teach.

I was a great teacher for beginners, because I really struggled both physically and mentally when I started practicing yoga. I taught yoga to stiff and stressed men, because I was one. I taught people to quit smoking because I smoked and gave it up successfully.

These are just the basics of what experience can add to your yoga teaching career. My wife went through my yoga teacher training and then became pregnant. She immediately learned how to teach pre-natal yoga and became a fabulous teacher as such. An older woman who taught at my studio had arthritis and is now teaching yoga to people that have arthritis.

The stories can go on. The gym teachers are teaching athletes, the elementary teachers are teaching their students, the nurses are teaching their patients, the physical therapist gives his clients complementary yoga exercises to do at home, the daycare specialist is teaching her toddlers, the reformed alcoholic is teaching in rehab, the college student is teaching her classmates, the tech-nerd is teaching his buddies who are stuck in front of the computer all day ...

It's a really simple formula:
Your experience + Yoga = New Students

What have you experienced that yoga has helped you resolve? Who are the people in your peer group? Answer these questions and you will be on your way to find a new group of people that are really interested in learning about yoga, but have never found a teacher they related to.

I have always said that training more yoga teachers is good for yoga. People that will come to your classes, read your books, and go to your lectures, will relate to *you* because of your background and experience. They might never come to the class of a much better known yoga teacher.

Once you integrate one area of expertise or experience with your yoga training you will find that it opens many doors; and that you will deepen your practice and understanding of yoga at the same time.

DON'T GIVE IN TO BOREDOM

"The most precious gift we can offer others is our presence. When mindfulness embraces those we love, they will bloom like flowers."
- Thich Nhat Hanh

Even though there seems to be an infinite number of yoga poses, every yoga teacher comes experiences the feeling of boredom at one point or another. Yoga is much like swimming. There are different swimming styles with different emphasis, but once you know them, you will only get better through repetition and practice.

Personally, I don't know how many times I have taught the shoulder stand, a simple forward bend, or guided people into relaxation. Having taught more than 6000 hours of yoga, I know I should probably be bored with teaching these same exercises, using the same wording, similar tone and hand gestures, but I'm not.

The reason that I have very seldom been bored with teaching is simple. I *decided* early on that I wouldn't become bored. I realized that I would be saying the same things over and over again, teaching same or similar postures, using the same tone of voice, spending hours and hours in the same rooms, and I vowed that I wouldn't let it get to me.

I have seen yoga teachers, almost in frenzy, looking for something new; new postures, breathing exercises, styles of yoga, teachers and so on. But what are they really searching for? *Escape from boredom.*

You escape boredom by being present! Experience each moment as new, and instead of dwelling on thoughts of repetition, see each student as new in this moment, remember to breathe deeply, serve your students and give them all your attention.

If you do this, you will guarantee two things. One is that you will never be bored. Two is that your students will return. People are energized in the presence of a person who is *ALL* there, who refuses to be distracted, and is completely present.

Total attention is the answer. It will transform teaching into a moving meditation.

LEARN TO INTERPRET AND TEACH THE PHILOSOPHICAL AND SPIRITUAL ASPECTS OF YOGA

"We commit to the goal and not to the means. The means may change as we evolve."
- Yogi Shanti Desai

Yoga has many philosophical and spiritual aspects to it. Some of them are applicable to everyday life, some are not. Through my reading, writings and teaching in the past years I have been doing my best to decipher the *yoga code* if you might, learn ways of presenting yogic philosophies to Western students through a variety of media, such as books, seminars, lectures, video and audio. I recently presented the core of yogic philosophy in modern context in a book titled *Living in the Spirit of Yoga: Take Yoga off the Mat and Into Everyday Life.*

I would like to encourage you to do something similar and present yoga philosophy to your students in a modern fashion. When you are reading the authentic yogic texts, sitting with a teacher, or talking to a student, think of ways to present this ancient material in a fashion that empowers your students; you can represent the practical aspects in everyday language and encourage your students to dig deeper instead of focusing only on the postures.

We are living in an information society and most people can now access the ancient yogic texts. But do they know how to live by them? Can they put the yogic ideas into practice within the context of their lives? Can you help steer them in that direction and help them make discoveries about themselves?

Maybe you can teach about the importance of relaxation, the power of concentration, and the different primal urges that drive us (action, passion and intellect), the need for compassion, the strength in humility, or the unending depths of the soul. There are plenty of topics to choose from.

Be non-judgmental and non-dogmatic; meet your students where *they are* and teach in accordance with your own experience.

Depending on your interests, and your students' interests and capacities, I urge you to teach and interpret more than the yoga postures. You will find it both rewarding and enriching in the safe space that you have created.

DON'T USE YOUR CLASSES FOR PERSONAL PRACTICE

*"Help your brothers boat across, and
your own will reach the shore."*
- Hindu proverb

I think most yoga teachers go through a period where they think it is great teaching yoga, simply because then they get to do so much of it; they get all the practice and become strong and flexible in the process. However, this should not be so. *Teaching should not be confused with personal practice.*

I have personally been to quite a few yoga classes where the teacher was more concerned with his own postures and breathing than with teaching the class, and I have heard many similar stories from my trainees. This is not a deadly sin, but it is a misunderstanding. A yoga teacher is not in the class for himself, he is there *for his students*, period.

My suggestion is that you learn to teach as much as you can without doing the exercises at the same time. Teach using your voice and body language.

Why do I emphasize this? That's an easy one, because of my own mistakes in this area. When I opened my yoga studio in Iceland in 2001, I didn't have much money, so I decided to be the *only* teacher in the studio for the first few months. The problem was that I had not trained myself to teach without doing the postures and I still viewed teaching as my personal practice. Well, you can imagine how well that experiment went. I started teaching in October and taught 22 classes a week, that's close to 90 classes a month! In January the following year I was seeing a chiropractor on a regular basis because I had almost ruined my back (go figure).

Primarily out of need, I started teaching without participating, and lo and behold, the attendance went up and the students started doing better.

One of the things that I love about teaching is the absolute focus one must bring to the class, being in the moment and honoring the task at hand. Students can feel that focus, and they want more once they recognize it. I have trained my voice, my body language and formulated my classes, so that even when I am having a bad day (which happens every now and then), I am better than average because of my training.

I emphasize this to all my teacher trainees, tell them they shouldn't rely on their bodies, only their voices if possible, and be able to teach from a wheelchair (if need be).

Disconnect your personal practice from your teaching and you will gain momentum in both areas.

DEEPEN YOUR PERSONAL PRACTICE

"Look well into thyself; there is a source which will always spring up if thou wilt always search there."
- Marcus Aurelius

Are you strong and flexible? If not, start there, and take care of your body. But if you are strong and flexible, ask yourself this: "How much stronger and more flexible can I become?" There is a point when you either begin maintaining the body and start digging deeper on the spiritual side, or you simply start injuring yourself because you are pushing your body too hard.

Yoga philosophy is pretty clear on all the areas we yogis and yoginis should work on in our practice. We should develop our mind and intellect (Gnana-Yoga), develop compassion and care (Bhakti-Yoga), serve through our actions and let go of the outcome (Karma-Yoga), and use the methods of physical and mental discipline to peel away the layers that cover our innermost being, the soul or Atman (Raja-Yoga). If you are only working on your body, you can easily see how much is being left out.

An integral or holistic practice includes all of the above, and perhaps more.

Think about how you are growing as a person through teaching. Are you training your mind? Are you becoming more compassionate? Are you attached to your surroundings, situation and ideas about yourself? What is your daily practice schedule like?

This chapter is not meant to make you feel guilty. But if you feel that there is something missing, and that you could evolve your yoga practice, be open to deepening it in some way, shape or form.

My teacher and friend, Yogi Shanti Desai, has a complaint about Western students. He says they stop showing up for class when they feel *guilty*, when they haven't done everything he instructed them to do, and when they haven't met their own standards. Yogi Shanti is such a dear man that he never pressures anyone to do anything, but he teaches the truth as he sees it, and that includes all the aspects of yoga, all the aspects of a human being. But he says that taking a guilt trip is not productive. He encourages his students to *be guilt free* while learning from their mistakes.

Jon Kabat-Zinn said that *wherever you go, there you are*. You can't outrun yourself. So if you have a practice, it will go with you, and if you don't, that truth about you will also go wherever you go.

Psychologist David Burns says that striving to be *perfect* means that you have something to hide, while striving for *progress* means that you are open to change and willing to explore the entirety of your being.

The poet Rumi said that one should keep knocking, and eventually a door would open; a door to both exquisite and divine experiences (in the poem *Sunrise Ruby*, when referring to personal spiritual practice).

Your personal practice is just that, your *personal* practice, and you should shape it based on your needs and the best available techniques and methods available at each time. Yoga is still open and evolving. There has been done excellent groundwork for us to work with and improve upon, but you can only improve something that you have already mastered.

ENCOURAGE GROWTH AND QUESTIONING

"He who asks a question is a fool for five minutes; he who does not ask a question remains a fool forever."
- Chinese proverb

One of the hallmarks of great teachers is that they rejoice when their students surpass them. Encouraging an atmosphere of questioning and inviting people to grow within your classroom isn't necessarily easy; which must explain why people who want to create cults or die hard followers discourage questioning in general. They would rather have people reciting their dogma than asking hard questions.

Face it, the guru who is never wrong, *doesn't exist*. A sincere soul, wanting to serve students, will encourage free thinking within the framework of a persistent practice. If you are sincere when you answer questions, then you can't go wrong, especially if you have learned to say "I don't know".

There is a principle related to this advice. If you want to debate mathematics, you must first be literate in the language of mathematics. People who aren't literate in mathematics will not be invited to discuss the harder mathematical problems, or will at least not be taken very seriously. The same is true with spiritual practice. To earn a right to sit at the table with the masters, and ask questions, you must practice.

When teaching you will soon see that the students who are practicing faithfully will ask better questions, which means that some of the questions that you will get from beginners will be questions of a lesser quality. I usually foster a safe space for growth and questioning by telling my students that there is no such thing as a stupid question.

In contradiction to that, I once studied with a teacher who used the phrase "You stupid idiot!" every time someone asked a question of a lesser quality. Even if this was done in a light hearted spirit, most of the time, it damaged the atmosphere of questioning. People became hesitant when he said "Any questions?"

Encouraging a questioning atmosphere will mean that you have to know what you are talking about, and it lessens your degree of control over people. But the benefits of questioning are obvious and it should be encouraged.

There is a difference between sincere questioning and trivial objections or quibbles. It seems that some people can't help themselves and are willing to try anything to show that they are smarter than the teacher. Be sure to keep your environment safe and controlled to a degree, not allowing other people to take over your class, but stay open to questions and remarks within a given timeframe when teaching or giving a talk.

One way to explain growth is as the ability to see things (internal and external) from a new or different *perspective*. When someone sets a new tone in a discussion, or offers a fresh point of view, it is in most cases wise to follow that train of thought, even if you are not familiar with the idea or point of view. When you are encouraging an atmosphere of growth, it entails that *you too* must be willing to *grow*.

USE MARKETING WITH A SERVICE ORIENTATION

"The aim of marketing is to know and understand the customer so well that the product or service fits him and sells itself."
- Peter F. Drucker

When I was first introduced to the *New Age* movement through my parents back in 1990, talk of money was an absolute *no, no*, and marketing was a sin (of sorts). This idea seemed to linger in the yoga teacher community in Iceland for a long time and by some I was considered a "sinner" for my marketing bravado.

Even though much of that thinking has changed over the years I find that most of my yoga teacher trainees have an unclear understanding of marketing and ways of monetizing their new found skills when they graduate. But if you don't market your-self, *there will be no students to create a safe space for.*

Here is what I believe to be true: *Marketing is a battle for attention.* When I began teaching yoga in 1998 a friend of mine said: "You know who your competition is? It's not other yoga teachers or yoga studios. No, it's the movies, the bars, and the inter-net, the entertainment industry as a whole, people's jobs and more. You need to get their *attention* in order to sell them the idea that yoga is good for them." And that is what I firmly believe until this day, that yoga is good for you (and me) and that if we work within the mindset of service to our fellow human beings, we *should* market our services.

The tools for marketing are constantly changing and will continue to do so for years to come. I am not talking about ruthless selling of a product in a win/lose scenario; but presenting your skills and services in a sincere manner. Marketing is really just about communication. Are you communicating to others about the benefits of yoga (within reason)?

I have never tried to force my ideas upon others. I have presented them on radio, through my books, my blogs, my TV shows, lectures, seminars and more, and in that way I have always given people the option to turn (me) off or walk away if they didn't like what I was presenting.

Remember the sentence from before? *"I am not going to like everyone, not everyone is going to like me, and that is perfectly OK."* You're going to need it when you are marketing yourself, because not everyone is going to like you, and that's OK.

Fear of failure and fear of rejection rule the actions of too many people, yoga teachers included. If you truly believe the essence of the yogic scriptures, then you must remember the words of *Krishna* from the *Bhagavad-Gita* as translated by Swami Prabhavananda and Christopher Isherwood:

Know this Atman
Unborn, undying,
Never ceasing,
Never beginning,
Deathless, birthless,
Unchanging for ever.
How can It die
The death of the body?

Knowing It birthless,

Knowing It deathless,
Knowing It endless,
For ever unchanging,
Dream not you do
The dead of a killer,
Dream not the power
Is yours to command it.

Worn-out garments
Are shed by the body:
Worn-out bodies
Are shed by the dweller
Within the body.
New bodies are donned
By the dweller, like garments.

Not wounded by weapons,
Not burned by fire,
Not dried by the wind,
Not wetted by water:
Such is the Atman,
Not dried, not wetted,
Not burned, not wounded,
Innermost element,
Everywhere, always,

Being of beings,
Changeless, eternal,
Forever and ever.

If you, through practice, introspection, commun-ion and contemplation, have experienced your real essence, *It* or *Atman*, then why should you be *con-trolled by fear*?

Even if many people think that marketing is the antithesis of spiritual practice, it seems to follow logic that if you want to positively affect other people, and offer them your services, then you simply *must* (in this densely populated world with an endless array of stimuli bombarding the ordinary citizen every day) be willing to market your ser-vices. By what means is up to you, but sitting at home thinking about why no one values your talents and services, and at the same time being afraid of rejection, is not a mirror image of your true Self. If you believe that we are all interconnected, that everything is Brahman (and if you don't know *Atman* and *Brahman* you should ask for your money back at the yoga teacher training), then the act of reaching out to another Soul, through all the means available to you, should not even be a thing to consider, just do it!

PRACTICE THE ETHICAL GUIDELINES OF YOGA

"A man's ethical behavior should be based effectually on sympathy, education, and social ties; no religious basis is necessary. Man would indeed be in a poor way if he had to be restrained by fear of punishment and hope of reward after death."
- Albert Einstein

As a yoga teacher you already know the *yamas* and the *niyamas*, also known as the ten commandments of yoga. There are two sides to yogic ethical guidelines, the *internal* and *external* aspects.

The internal aspect is connected to the small still voice within. If you are in line with the ethical guidelines you will have less anxiety, fear and restlessness.

The external aspect affects your immediate surroundings and pertains to your job as a yoga teacher and is closely related to ethical concerns in general, many of which try to answer the question: "How should we treat other people?"

In this chapter I don't want to pretend that I know all the ways in which to interpret the ethical guidelines within a modern framework. I just want to encourage you to read the *yamas* and *niyamas* carefully with the external, and especially the teaching aspect in mind.

If you contemplate the ethical guidelines, ask yourself: "How would I treat my students if I followed these ethics."

Following ethical standards can be hard, especially if they are represented as rules, punishable in a cruel afterlife. From that standpoint ethics become a burden and ignite all sorts of inner battles and inconsistencies, eventually leading to psychological problems (ask any good therapist).

If, on the other hand, ethics are represented as guidelines, or even better, a version of *how a master of life would live*, then ethics can be very useful in the betterment of one's own character, igniting a will to change and better serve the surrounding world.

Even if ethics have an external side to them, they are mostly internal in nature. In order to treat people a certain way, you have to be willing to treat yourself in the same manner. Gandhi wisely said that peace of mind can be found through consistency between thought, word and deed. If you *think* one thing, *say* another and then *do* the third, you are in conflict with yourself.

Again I remind you of the idea of improvement over perfection. The yogic scriptures surely paint a picture of perfection, and perfection can be your *aim*, but I have sad stories about myself and others who have entered "premature holiness" with unpleasant consequences.

If in doubt, just be nice!

INFUSE YOGA WITH MODERN APPROACHES TO CREATE THE YOGA OF THE FUTURE

"Do not believe anything on the mere authority of teachers or priests. Accept as true and as the guide to your life only that which accords with your own reason and experience, after thorough investigation. Accept only that which contributes to the well-being of yourself and others."
- Buddha

One of the things that troubled me after a few years of studying yoga was the incessant focus on the past. The yogis of old were said to have lived in constant bliss, and our world was said to have turned into total rubbish to put it mildly. But when comparing this worldview with the view of many of today's leading scientists I don't believe that to be true anymore.

I believe that many yoga practices have stood the test of time, and in the area of self-exploration, within the confines of the mind and beyond, we as a species can be very grateful to the preceding yogis and yoginis.

But I also believe in the betterment of the future. I would agree with Hans Rosling when he says that he is neither a negativist nor a positivist, but a *possibilist* (which is a belief in possibilities).

I see possibilities in the fact that the human race hasn't annihilated itself even if it has had the power to do so, that people are generally living longer than ever before, and that there are brilliant minds working on the world's most pressing problems in every continent. I am a follower of better education, better health care, and better standards of living for all, but at the same time I believe in better quality of thinking and human growth potential, which the ancient practices of yoga can help us realize.

I have been reading and talking about the marriage of Eastern and Western thought for over twenty years now and I genuinely believe that we are glacially inching in that direction, but there is a lot of work to be done. The citizens of the world face enormous problems and we can be solution oriented or fatalistic. I prefer solution orientation.

I believe that we can bring the yogic clarity of thinking to everything we do. We should not run away from the world, but live in it as loving servants without becoming too attached to the outcome. I haven't completely mastered *the way* of uniting East and West, uniting sense and soul, science and spirituality, balancing *Prakriti* and *Purusha*, matter and spirit; but I am willing to believe in the possibility. I am willing to struggle with it, entertain the notion, and try to put the idea into action, thus creating a safer space for all of us.

Yoga philosophy is vast and there are numerous practices to choose from. I would like to enlist you, the yoga teacher, as a fellow *possibilist*, and ask you to remain open to new ways of linking the ancient and modern, and when you do find new ways, share them with others, you are a teacher after all.

CONCLUSION:
ALL ABOUT SERVICE

"The best way to find yourself is to lose yourself in the service of others."
- Mohandas Gandhi

I started writing this book on the airplane on my way to a new life in the USA earlier this year. I wanted to offer other yoga teachers some of the experience I have gathered through the years. The book is short, to the point, and covers everything that I wanted to say. I hope that you, the yoga teacher, have benefitted from reading it. You may not agree with everything I have written, and that's OK, but I hope that I have at least gotten you to think about your role as a yoga teacher and your commitment to your students. My goal is simple. I want to help you serve your students. That's it. If I have succeeded please contact me through *www.gudjonbergmann.com* and let me know.

Gudjon Bergmann, 2010

www.ingramcontent.com/pod-product-compliance
Lightning Source LLC
Chambersburg PA
CBHW062054280526
45788CB00003B/1224